Prostate Health

by

Georgina Cyr

Certified Herbalist, Nutritional Health Consultant

Table of Contents

Prostate Health

If you are a man and not sure what your prostate is or what it does, you are not alone. This is sometimes embarrassing and difficult to talk about. If you are one of those men, or if you would like to know more about prevention and early diagnosis, this book is for you. Your life could depend upon it. If you are a woman reading this book, your partner is a lucky man. Your support is a valuable commodity.

What is the Prostate?

The prostate is a small little gland that sits beneath the bladder, behind the scrotal sac. It is in the shape of a little donut, the size of a walnut shell and through the prostate is the urethra.

Dietary prevention, fitness and early diagnosis are the key to long term prostate health. Every year there are thousands of men who are treated for inflamed prostate, which in most cases, could have been prevented.

Over fifty percent of men in their sixties and ninety percent of men in their seventies or older develop symptoms of an enlarged prostate.

Most prostate problems are caused by an enlarged prostate. As a man ages, the chance of him having this problem increases. An enlarged prostate means infection not cancer. Common prostate problems are BPH (benign prostatic hyperplasia), prostate enlargement, and Prostatis.

The prostate expands and contracts like a small balloon. An orgasm is the result of the contraction. When the prostate fills with semen until it can't hold any more, it ejaculates and contracts until it shrinks down again. It should be soft and have elasticity like a balloon, so that it can swell and shrink easily. If the prostate loses its elasticity, it can swell and not have the ability to shrink again, continue to be swollen and develop an inflamed condition, called Prostatis. It can then go onto becoming enlarged, which is called Benign Prostatis Hypertrophy, BPH.

Prostatis

Prostatis means the prostate might be irritated or inflamed. Inflammation is an indication that the body is either repairing an injury or fighting infection.

Signs of an inflamed or irritated prostate are:

- Fever
- Burning feeling when you urinate
- Urinating more frequently
- Feeling tired

Some kinds of prostates are caused by bacteria. If you have bacterial prostates the doctor can determine this by looking at a sample of your urine through a microscope. If bacteria are found, the doctor can give you an antibiotic to kill the bacteria.

If there is no bacterial found and the doctor has ruled out a possible problem with kidney stones or cancer, he may determine that you have nonbacterial prostatis. Your doctor will then be able to recommend a treatment that's right for you.

BPH, Prostate Enlargement

The prostate gland grows and doubles in size from birth to age twenty-five. It stops growing then until about age fifty where it continues to grow again until about age seventy. This is called benign prostatic hyperplasia. This non-cancerous enlargement is part of the normal maturation process in all men. Enlarged prostate is not life threatening, nor is it cancerous. It can however, if left untreated, lead to other problems such as kidney damage, bladder stones, urinary retention, and urinary infections.

The prostate gland grows through these two phases because of changes in the hormonal levels. When a man reaches the age of about fifty, the levels of testosterone and estrogen change, with the levels of estrogen increasing in relation to the testosterone. It is thought that the increase in estrogen promotes cell growth in the prostate gland.

As the prostate grows it can put excess pressure on the urethra, a small tube that carries the semen and urine. With the increase in pressure the urethra can become pinched. This can lead to embarrassing and painful symptoms such as erectile dysfunction, urinary hesitancy and painful urination. It is important to see your doctor for treatment as if left untreated they can require surgery.

Signs of BPH

- Needing to urinate frequently
- A weak stream of urine
- Trouble starting a urine stream even though you have an urgency to urinate
- A small amount of urine each time
- Leaking or dribbling urine
- Feeling like to have to go even though you've just finished urinating
- Blood in your urine

Bacteria

The prostate sits over the sigmoid area of the colon, where fecal matter is held until elimination. Fatty and fried foods tend to weaken the colon wall by accumulating with bacteria which could pass through the colon wall to the prostate. 96% of all prostate cancer is on the side of the prostate that sits next to the colon wall. Washing your anus after fecal expulsion also helps to stop bacteria from multiplying in the anal area.

Other Causes

In most healthy people, urine in the bladder is sterile, containing no negative bacteria or other infectious organisms. The tube that carries urine from the bladder out of the body (urethra) in a healthy body usually contains no bacteria. If an infection occurs anywhere along the urinary tract, it is called a urinary tract infection (UTI).

UTIs are usually classified as upper or lower depending on where they occur along the urinary tract. Infections of the urethra (urethritis) or bladder (cystitiscan be classified as lower UTIs. Doctors usually consider prostate infections to be lower UTIs). Infections of the kidneys (pyelonephritis are often classified as upper UTIs, however, infection can occur in both areas.

The organisms that can cause infection usually through a man's urethra at the tip of the penis or the opening of a woman's urethra. The infection runs up the urethra to the bladder, or kidneys, or sometimes both. It is possible for the infection to come through the bloodstream as well with the cause usually being excessive toxicity, often due to issues with the colon intestines.

UTIs are often caused by bacteria, although viruses, fungi, and parasites can infect the urinary tract as well.
Many UTIs are caused by bacteria from the intestine or vagina.

Bacteria: Bacterial infections are very commonly caused by Ecoli. Women are the most affected by bacterial UTIs, because the urethra in men is longer until they reach the age of 50 where both sexes seems to be more equally affected.
Kidneys stones make the Urethra more susceptible to UTIs.
Some of the factors that can create Bacterial Urinary Tract Infections

- Sexual intercourse
- Infection in the bloodstream (septicemia)
- Infection of the heart valves (infective endocarditis)

- herpes simplex virus type 2 (HSV-2)
- Fungi or yeast, can infect the urinary tract.
- Candida Albicans is the most common cause of urinary tract infections

Less Common are:
- Parasites
- Trichomoniasis –(a sexually transmitted parasite)
- Schistosomiasis, (a worm type parasite)
- Filariasis,(a threadworm infections causing swelling involving the lymphatic system)

What tests might my Doctor recommend?

PSA Testing

It does not necessarily mean that a man has prostate cancer if he has an elevated PSA. There are other conditions other than cancer that can cause the elevation. An infection or a benign enlargement of the prostate can result in higher than normal PSA levels.

It's important to note that a PSA test is not always foolproof. False negative test results can occur when prostate cancer is present, even though the number is in the normal range. It has also been found that no cancer was present even though the PSA level was high. This is known as a false positive test result.

It has become a controversial issue whether the PSA test should be used to screen men for prostate cancer as it is not clear whether the benefits outweigh the risks of follow up testing and treatments.

A PSA test may detect small cancers that would never be life threatening to a man and then he would be put at risk from complications from treatment that was unnecessary.

Most men die with prostate cancer but not from it. They never knew they even had the cancer, because the prostate keeps it contained. It never leaks out…unless because of outside influences, it spreads into the blood.

A biopsy may cause harmful side effects such as infection and bleeding. Surgery and radiation may cause erectile dysfunction and incontinence. It is important to take the benefits, risks and treatments into account when considering whether or not to undertake prostate cancer screening.

I would like to include reference to a study done by Smith DS, Humphrey PA, Catalona WJ. The early detection of prostate carcinoma with prostate specific antigen: The Washington University experience. *Cancer* 1997; 80(9):1853–1856.

"The early detection of prostate carcinoma with prostate specific antigen: The Washington University experience. *Cancer* 1997; 80(9):1853–1856PSA test results show the level of PSA detected in the blood. These results are usually reported as nanograms of PSA per milliliter (ng/mL) of blood. In the past, most doctors considered a PSA level below 4.0 ng/mL as normal.

In one large study, however, prostate cancer was diagnosed in 15.2 percent of men with a PSA level at or below 4.0 ng/mL (2). Fifteen percent of these men, or approximately 2.3 percent overall, had high-grade cancers (2).

In another study, 25 to 35 percent of men who had a PSA level between 4.1 and 9.9 ng/mL and who underwent a prostate biopsy were found to have prostate cancer, meaning that 65 to 75 percent of the remaining men did not have prostate cancer."

Experts recommend that the PSA test should be combined with a digital rectal exam for best results.

Digital Rectal Exam

The Digital Rectal Exam cannot diagnose prostate cancer however it is used to determine if further testing is necessary. It has been recommended that all men over the age of 50 have a Digital Rectal Exam.

In this exam a doctor inserts a gloved, lubricated finger into a man's rectum in order to feel the prostate. If the doctor finds a roughness and irregular unevenness to the tissue, prostate issues might be suspected. An enlarged prostate that is not cancerous will likely still feel smooth.

MRI Scan

A magnetic resonance imaging (MRI) scan is a computerized picture that can show detailed, images of the inner body. This scan makes it possible to see a clear picture of the prostate gland.

Ultrasound

An ultrasound is usually performed by passing a sensor over the surface of a person's body. The high-frequency sound waves bounce off organs and body structures and produce a computerized image. When the prostate is examined, a tube is inserted into the rectum. This carries the sound waves to the nearby prostate and an image is produced.

Biopsy

When a biopsy is taken, a fine needle is used to take a small sample of tissue. It is then examined under a microscope to see if there are any malignant cells.

The biopsy could be performed in various ways and it is always a good idea to ask the doctor ahead of time what the procedure will involve, whether medication will be given to prevent any discomfort, and if there are any risks involved.

Some possible complications may include, but are not limited to, the following:

- Bruising and discomfort at the biopsy site.
- Prolonged bleeding from the biopsy site.
- Infection near the biopsy site.
- Difficulty urinating.

What can you do to promote Prostate Health?

Healthy Eating

Developing good eating habits goes a long way to staying healthy. It is important to make sure we eat healthy foods that contain antioxidants.

Antioxidants are substances that are capable of counteracting the damaging, but normal, effects of the process of oxidation in tissue. Oxidation is the name of the process your body goes through when the heat and energy your body needs are produced through the metabolizing of glucose and fats. Antioxidants are nutrients (vitamins and minerals) as well as enzymes (proteins in your body that assist in chemical reactions). They are believed to play a role in preventing the development of cancer.

Food remains the smart choice for where to obtain your antioxidants. Studies consistently demonstrate that for optimum health, you should eat at least five servings of vegetables everyday as part of a balanced diet.

Herbs for Prostate Health

Herbs have a powerful effect if you are working to keep your prostate healthy and clean. Saw Palmetto berry has been known to effectively diminish inflammation, pain and enlargement of the prostate. It is also thought to have a mild aphrodisiac effect as well as increasing sexual vitality.

Pygeum africanum , an herb from an African evergreen tree, has been shown to reduce prostatic enlargement and inflammation. It has many natural chemicals that have anti-inflammatory effects on the body.

Antioxidants

Some of the antioxidants that our bodies need are in Vitamin C, Vitamin E, Selenium, Manganese, Zinc, and Beta-Carotene.

Vitamin C

Vitamin C, also known as ascorbic acid, is a water-soluble vitamin. It attacks free radicals that are inside your cells. Vitamin C works with vitamin E to destroy free radicals. Good choices of foods to find Vitamin C in are broccoli, cantaloupe, citrus fruits (grapefruit, oranges), leafy green vegetables, peppers, potatoes, strawberries and tomatoes.

Vitamin E

Vitamin E is found in almonds, avocado, leafy green vegetables, olives, seeds, vegetable oils, walnuts and wheat germ.

Selenium

Selenium is a trace element. It is a mineral that we need to consume in only very small quantities, but without which we could not survive. Selenium is found in beef, brazil nuts, brown rice, chicken, pork, seafood and whole wheat bread.

Manganese and Zinc

Similar to selenium, the minerals **manganese** and **zinc** are trace elements that form an essential part of various antioxidant enzymes.

Manganese is found in brown rice, chard, cloves (dried, ground), collard greens, garbanzo beans, kale, maple syrup, mustard greens, oats (whole grain), pineapple, raspberries, romaine lettuce, rye (whole grain), spelt grains (cooked), spinach (boiled) and Tempeh (cooked).

Zinc is found in beef, dairy products, lima beans, nuts (cashews, almonds, pecans), oysters, peas, pumpkin seeds, seafood, and turkey.

Beta-carotene

Beta-carotene is a water-soluble vitamin. It is also excellent at scavenging free radicals. Beta-carotene is found in apricots, cantaloupe, kale, mangoes, papaya, peppers, pumpkin, spinach, squash, carrots and sweet potatoes.

Phytochemicals

It is also important for a person to eat foods containing phytochemicals in order to maintain good health. Phytochemicals are chemical compounds that occur naturally in plants. The term is generally used to refer to those chemicals that *may* affect health, but are not yet established as essential nutrients.

Following are some of the phytochemicals and what foods you can find them in.

Allyl sulfides are found in chives, garlic, leeks and onions.

Carotenoids are found in carrots, kale, spinach, tomatoes and watermelon.

Curcumin is found in tumeric.

Flavonoids are found in apples, blackberries, cherries, cranberries, grapefruit, grapes, raspberries and strawberries.

Quercetin acts as an antihistamine and has anti-inflammatory properties, which may be helpful in relieving the pain of an inflamed prostate. Foods rich in Quercetin are: apples, black and green tea, broccoli, cherries, citrus fruits, honey and sap (including the type from eucalyptus and tea tree flowers), leafy green vegetables, onions, raspberries, red grapes and red wine.

Glutathione is found in green leafy vegetables.

Indoles are found in bok choy, broccoli, brussel sprouts, cabbage and cauliflower.

Isoflavones are found in legumes (peas, soybeans).

Isothiocyanates are found in bok choy, broccoli, brussel sprouts, cauliflower and cabbage.

Lignans are found in seeds (flax, sunflower)

Monoterpenes are found in cherries, citrus fruit peels and nuts.

Phytic acid is found in legumes and whole grains.

Phenols, polyphenols, phenolic compounds are found in blackberries, blueberries, cherries, cranberries, grapefruit, grapes, raspberries an tea (green and black).

Saponins are found in beans and legumes.

The Importance of Essential Fatty Acids

It is important to know the difference between good fats and bad fats as it is believed that rates of cancer are tied to imbalances in our diets between good and bad fats.

Some fats are damaged because of the heat used in the refining process. These are hydrogenated, artificially hardened and saturated. Examples of these would be shortenings and margarines.
Even if they are from vegetable sources and cholesterol free, they are still loaded with dangerous trans-fatty acids. Our body doesn't recognize them as food because they have become like plastic.

All saturated fats are bad for us. This would include the fats from animal products, such as red meat, pork etc.

Good fats compete with the bad fats in our body. The good fats raise your High Density Lipoprotein (HDL) or "good cholesterol". It is important to eat enough good fats so that they can grab onto the bad fats and remove them from our body. They escort the bad fats to the liver where the bad fat is broken down and excreted.

The good news is that polyunsaturated fats are great for us. They provide the essential fatty acids the body requires for good health and are the omega-3 oils.

Omegas 3's also really help with reducing inflammation and assisting the whole body to be healthier overall. EFAs support the cardiovascular, reproductive, immune, and nervous systems. The human body needs EFAs to manufacture and repair cell membranes, enabling the cells to obtain optimum nutrition and expel harmful waste products. A primary function of EFAs is the production of prostaglandins, which regulate body functions such as heart rate, blood pressure, blood clotting, and play a role in immune function by regulating and reducing inflammation and encouraging the body to fight infection.

Essential Fatty Acids (EFAs) are necessary fats that humans cannot synthesize, and must be obtained through diet. There are two families of EFAs: Omega-3 and Omega-6.

Omega-9 is necessary yet "non-essential" because the body can manufacture a modest amount on its own, provided essential EFAs are present.

Omega-3 fatty acids are derived from Linolenic Acid, Omega-6 from Linoleic Acid, and Omega-9 from Oleic Acid.

Omega-3 (Linolenic Acid) is found in the following foods:

- avocados
- Brazil nuts
- canola oil (cold-pressed and unrefined)
- fish – salmon, mackerel, sardines, anchovies, albacore tuna.
- flaxseed oil (flaxseed oil has the highest linolenic content of any food)
- flaxseeds, flaxseed meal
- hempseed oil, hempseeds
- pumpkin seeds
- sesame seeds

- dark leafy green vegetables (kale, spinach, mustard greens, collards, etc.)
- soybean oil - non gmo
- walnuts
- wheat germ oil

Although recent research is showing that most of us are lacking in Omega 3s and do not need to supplement with Omega 6 and 9 – here are a list of foods that have Omega 6 and 9.

It is always best to speak with your health profession in regards to your own bodies individual needs.

Omega-6 (Linoleic Acid) is found in foods such as:

- black currant seed oil
- borage oil
- chestnut oil
- chicken
- evening primrose oil
- flaxseed oil, flaxseeds, flaxseed meal
- grapeseed oil
- hempseed oil, hempseeds
- olive oil
- olives
- pumpkin seeds
- pine nuts
- pistachio nuts

- sunflower seeds (raw)

Omega-9 (Oleic Acid) is found in:

- almonds
- avocados
- cashews
- hazelnuts
- macadamia nuts
- olive oil (extra virgin or virgin)
- olives
- peanuts
- pecans
- pistachio nuts
- sesame oil

Eating Tips

- Raw nuts are a better source of EFA's than roasted nuts. High heat, light, and oxygen destroy the essential fatty acids.
- Use Flaxseed, coconut oil and extra virgin olive oils on your vegetables instead of butter or margarine.
- Do not use flaxseed oil when cooking.
- Use extra virgin olive oil or coconut oil or grape seed oil for cooking oil, as they withstand high heat well.
- Eat nuts and seeds instead of potato chips and corn chips
- Broil, bake, steam, poach or roast food whenever possible.
- Instead of butter, margarine, or cream cheese, top your bread with jelly, jam, coconut oil, apple butter or hummus.
- Use hummus, garlic, or salsa on baked potatoes.
- For sandwich spread, instead of mayonnaise, use mustard, or mango chutney
- Use lots of garlic, onions, lemon juice and herbs in cooking.
- Eat lots of vegetables
- Eat less red meat
- Eat less saturated fats
- Drink more water
- Avoid caffeine
- Limit alcohol
- Avoid tobacco

Exercise

More and more research has shown that changes to your lifestyle can lead to prostate cancer prevention. Regular exercise for at least thirty minutes a day for three days per week is essential for prostate health.

If you are unsure if you really need to exercise, check out the other benefits shown below. There are many reasons to exercise.

Benefits of Exercise

- Give you more energy
- Help you sleep better
- Make you feel happier
- Reduce your risk of cancer and heart disease
- Helps to relieve anxiety and depression
- Lose weight
- Increase bone density
- Makes your lungs and heart stronger

The hardest part of exercise is getting motivated to start. Now that you know that it can help to keep your prostate healthy, you know you have a good reason to exercise. Remind yourself that this is necessary for you to maintain your goal of good health.

Cardio exercise strengthens the lungs and heart, burns calories and increases endurance. This includes a wide range of activities like aerobics, cycling, walking and running, dancing and swimming.

Strength training is another form of exercise that works the body in a different way than cardio. With strength training, you lift weights to strengthen the connective tissue, bones and muscles.

Keeping Yourself Flexible

Stretching is one of the most important exercises for keeping us agile as we age. The bonus is that it's relaxing and feels good. Stretching is also important to do after each workout.

Stretch a minimum of two or three days a week. Stretching shouldn't hurt so make sure you only stretch within your range of motion. Hold each stretch for about 15 – 30 seconds.

If you don't like to exercise alone, check out your local stretching, yoga and Pilates classes you could join. This is also a great way to keep you motivated and continue with your exercise program.

The Simple Things

Sometimes it's the really simple things that can help us to stay fit. Next time you park your car at a mall try parking just a bit further away from the door than you usually do. Take the stairs instead of the escalator or elevator. Take a walk after work or if you live close to work, walk instead of drive. Take your dog for a walk. All of these little things add up to help us maintain good health.

The best exercise for you to do is doing something you already like. Think about things you like to do and make that part of your daily activity.

Tips

- When you begin your exercise program, make sure you start slowly. If you do too much too soon you may find excuses to not continue such as being too sore, too stiff etc.

- Make sure you have shoes suitable for the activity you have chosen.

- Drink plenty of water.

- Be nice to yourself. If you're tired or ache all over, give yourself a day off from exercising to recover.

Prostate Exercises

Keigle - Squeeze your anus and testicles – squeeze hard, lift, and hold for a few seconds, release. Do five exercises three times a day or more.

Deer Exercise – rub hands together briskly with clothes off. Rub till hands get warm. Take your two long fingers, push on the bulb behind your scrotal sac, with your testicles sitting in the palm of your hand, squeeze your anus, lift and hold, and with your other hand, put it between your belly button and pubic bone and rub the area for 81 rubs. Then start over with the other hand and do 81 rubs. Do this twice a day. It increases the circulation to the prostate to promote healing. (Doing this before sex prevents premature ejaculation for most men.)

Exercise is extremely important…splits and butterfly type exercises work on the prostate area, strengthening the perineal floor.

Prostate Massage and Check

Use Vitamin E or K Y Jelly…do not use anything petroleum based. After your shower when your bowels are empty, enter your anal canal with your long finger, go as far as you can straight in and turn towards your pubic bone, you will feel the round bulb of your prostate. Check to see if it is hard, swollen or sensitive. Gently massage it to keep it soft and pliable. After your prostate massage, does it burn when you urinate? Is there blood in your urine? Is it unusually sensitive? If the answers to any of these are "yes" be sure to see your doctor for a thorough examination and tests.

Kidneys

It's important to take care of the kidneys as they are in charge of the reproductive organ. Good foods to eat for healthy kidneys are black beans, kidney beans, aduki beans, seaweed, millet, celery, parsley, carrots, asparagus and watermelon.

Helpful herbs are bee pollen, royal jelly, chlorophyll, saw palmetto berries, damaina, yohimbe. There is a men's formula by Flora that is especially good for the kidneys and prostate. It is also important to eat foods that contain Vitamins C Vitamin E and Zinc.

Kidney Massage

You can also massage your kidneys. Gently rub your kidneys, then make hollow fists and gently tap your kidneys, tap and rub, tap and rub.

Prostate Cancer

Prostate Cancer is one of the most common forms of cancer. Many men will develop prostate cancer by the time they are seventy. The cancer cells grow slowly and can remain inside the prostate gland for many years.

If you are diagnosed….what can you do?

There is a fearful silence that usually surrounds a man when he is diagnosed with prostate cancer. It is a subject that is usually not talked about and can make one feel totally alone in the struggle. Men are embarrassed to talk about subjects such as impotence and incontinence so many men go through the journey feeling lonely and fearful.

It is common for a man to go through the stages of fear, anger and then fighting back. Use anger as a tool to move ahead and improve what you can. The anger comes from questions such as Why me? Why has it changed my life so drastically? And why have things been taken away from me?

It is important for a man to have a good support group and a good sense of humor. Laughing is good for the immune system. A good diet and exercise are essential for recovery.

Hormones are sometimes used to treat cancer and this usually causes impotence and loss of libido. However, the upside of this is that when you go off of the hormones, the effects are reversible and life can be normal again.

I hope this information has been helpful. Please see your health professional for further information.

Light Blessings
Georgina Cyr